Intermittent Fasting

The Ultimate Beginner's Guide to Intermittent Fasting, Lose Weight & Live Healthy

Table of Contents

Introduction

I want to thank you and congratulate you for downloading the book, "Intermittent Fasting: The Ultimate Beginner's Guide to Intermittent Fasting, Lose Weight & Live Healthy".

This book contains proven steps and strategies on how to undertake intermittent fasting.

Intermittent Fasting (IF) refers to dietary eating patterns that involve not eating or severely restricting calories for a prolonged period. There are many different subgroups of intermittent fasting each with individual variation in the duration of the fast; some for hours, others for the day(s). This has become an extremely popular topic in the science community due to all of the potential benefits of fitness and health that are being discovered.

Fasting or periods of voluntary abstinence from food has been practiced throughout the world for ages. Intermittent fasting with the goal of improving health relatively new. Intermittent fasting involves restricting intake of food for a set period and does not include any changes to the actual foods you are eating. Currently, the most common IF protocols are a daily 16 hour fast and fasting for a whole day, one or two days per week. Intermittent fasting could be considered a natural eating pattern that humans are built to implement, and it traces all the way back to our paleolithic hunter-gatherer ancestors. The current model of a planned program of intermittent fasting could potentially help improve many aspects of health from body composition to longevity and aging. Although IF goes against the norms of our culture and common daily routine, the science may be pointing to less meal frequency and more time fasting as the optimal alternative to the normal breakfast, lunch, and dinner model. Here are two common myths that pertain to intermittent fasting.

Myths

Myth 1 - You Must Eat 3 Meals Per Day:

This "rule" that is common in Western society was not developed based on evidence for improved health, but was adopted as the common pattern for settlers and eventually became the norm. Not only is there a lack of scientific rationale in the 3 meal-a-day model, recent studies may be showing fewer meals and more fasting to be optimal for human health. One study showed that one meal a day with the same amount of daily calories is better for weight loss and body composition than 3 meals per day. This finding is a basic concept that is extrapolated into intermittent fasting and those choosing to do IF may find it best only to eat 1-2 meals per day.

Myth 2 - You Need Breakfast, It's The Most Important Meal of The Day:

Many false claims about the absolute need for a daily breakfast have been made. The most common claims being "breakfast increases your metabolism" and "breakfast decreases food intake later in the day." These claims have been refuted and studied over a 16 week period with results showing that skipping breakfast did not decrease metabolism and it did not increase food intake at lunch and dinner. It is still possible to do intermittent fasting protocols while still eating breakfast, but some people find it easier to eat a late breakfast or skip it altogether, and this common myth should not get in the way.

Thanks again for downloading this book, I hope you enjoy it!

Chapter 1: Types of Intermittent Fasting

Intermittent fasting comes in various forms, and each may have a specific set of unique benefits. Each form of intermittent fasting has variations in the fasting-to-eating ratio. The benefits and effectiveness of these different protocols may differ on an individual basis, and it is important to determine which one is best for you. Factors that may influence which one to choose include health goals, daily schedule/routine, and current health status. The most common types of IF are alternate day fasting, time-restricted feeding, and modified fasting.

ALTERNATE DAY FASTING:

This approach involves alternating days of absolutely no calories (from food or beverage) with days of free feeding and eating whatever you want.

This plan has been shown to help with weight loss, improve blood cholesterol and triglyceride (fat) levels, and improve markers of inflammation in the blood.

The main downfall with this form of intermittent fasting is that it is the most difficult to stick with because of the reported hunger during fasting days.

MODIFIED FASTING - 5:2 DIET

Modified fasting is a protocol with programmed fasting days, but the fasting days do allow for some food intake. 20-25% of, normal calories are allowed to be consumed on fasting days; so if you normally consume 2000 calories on regular eating days, you would be allowed 400-500 calories on fasting days. The 5:2 part of this diet refers to the ratio of non-fasting to fasting days. Soon this regimen, you would normally eat for 5 consecutive days, then fast or restrict calories to 20-25% for 2 consecutive days.

This protocol is great for weight loss, body composition, and may also benefit the regulation of blood sugar, lipids, and inflammation. Studies have shown the 5:2 protocol to be effective for weight loss, improve/lower inflammation markers in the blood (3), and show signs trending improvements in insulin resistance. In animal studies, this modified fasting 5:2 diet resulted in decreased fat, decreased hunger hormones (leptin), and increased levels of a protein responsible for improvements in fat burning and blood sugar regulation (adiponectin).

The modified 5:2 fasting protocol is easy to follow and has a small number of negative side effects which included hunger, low energy, and some irritability when beginning the program. Contrary to this, however, studies have also noted improvements such as reduced tension, less anger, less fatigue, improvements in self-confidence, and a more positive mood.

TIME-RESTRICTED FEEDING

If you know anyone that has said they are doing intermittent fasting, odds are it is in the form of time-restricted feeding. This is a type of intermittent fasting that is used daily, and it involves only consuming calories during a small portion of the day and fasting for the remainder. Daily fasting intervals in time-restricted feeding may range from 12-20 hours, with the most common method being 16/8 (fasting for 16 hours, consuming calories for 8). For this protocol, the time of day is not important as long as you are fasting for a consecutive period and only eating in your allowed period. For example, on a 16/8 time-restricted feeding program one person may eat their first meal at 7 AM and last meal at 3 PM (fast from 3PM-7AM), while another person may eat their first meal at 1 PM and last meal at 9 PM (fast from 9PM-1PM). This protocol is meant to be performed every day over long periods of time and is very flexible as long as you are staying within the fasting/eating window(s).

Time-Restricted feeding is one of the easiest to follow methods of intermittent fasting. Using this along with your daily work and sleep schedule may help achieve optimal metabolic function. Time-restricted feeding is a great program to follow for weight loss and body composition improvements as well as some other overall health benefits. The few human trials that were conducted noted significant reductions in weight, reductions in fasting blood glucose, and improvements in cholesterol with no changes in perceived tension, depression, anger, fatigue, or confusion. Some other preliminary results from animal studies showed time-restricted feeding to protect against obesity, high insulin levels, fatty liver disease, and inflammation.

The easy application and promising results of time-restricted feeding could make it an excellent option for weight loss and chronic disease prevention/management. When implementing this protocol, it may be good, to begin with, a lower fasting-to-eating ratio like 12/12 hours and eventually work your way up to 16/8 hours.

Chapter 2: Keys to Understanding Intermittent Fasting

With intermittent fasting becoming more and more popular as a weight-loss and health management diet, it is important to understand how to set it up; here are three keys to making sure that you can get involved in an intermittent fasting lifestyle as soon as possible.

- Intermittent fasting doesn't need to be a short-term approach to dieting and is in fact much more successful as a genuine lifestyle choice. The first decision to make therefore is how to adopt a fast to YOUR life. Remember that the fast can be anywhere from 16 hours to several days in length depending on exactly what you are trying to accomplish. The two approaches that are perhaps easiest to set up are an alternating day (24 hours) fast/eat cycle or a 16/8 cycle.

- When do I workout? This question is key. Diet is with doubt the most important factor in weight-loss and good health, but to get the best out of an intermittent fast, the re-feed should coincide with your workout. Personally, I have had success with a fast from 8 Pm until the next day at lunch and an early afternoon training session. All the food that I am taking in around my workout is being used for fuel and to repair muscle rather than being stocked as body-fat.

- What do I want to accomplish with intermittent fasting? Is your aim fat-loss, muscle gain, improved health or a combination of all three? You can begin to distinguish exactly how long your fast should be and what quantity of food you should be eating during the eating "window."

Chapter 3: Benefits of Intermittent Fasting

Weight loss and muscle gain are the most visible benefits of fasting. Nevertheless, there are numerous benefits linked with intermittent fasting beyond fat burning and muscle gain. In the old days, fasting periods were referred to as detoxification, purification and other synonyms for cleansing the body. The primary idea is to refrain from eating food for a precise period. Also, intermittent fasting is very different from dieting, which is difficult and can be expensive too.

There are many benefits of intermittent fasting, the most important of which are the following:

• Intermittent fasting, when paired with clean, organic, nutritious food eaten in moderation and the bonus of physical activity, can result in steady, consistent weight loss that stays off!

• Maintenance and potential gain of lean muscle mass

• Improved metabolism, which is beneficial to Brain Health, Metabolism is the name for the crucial chemical reactions that happen in your cells.

• Improved Ketone production. Ketone is a chemical that protects the brain when there is a decrease of available glucose.

• Improves appetite control – Intermittent Fasting allows you to discern between mental and physical hunger

• May reduce symptoms of depression by regulating insulin and blood sugar levels.

• Enhances performance on memory tests in the elderly

• Reduces Oxidative stress, damage, and inflammation in the body

• Hormonal Rebalancing – Insulin Levels and Insulin Resistance; Leptin; Ghrelin Also, Human Growth Hormone increases and facilitates fat burning and muscle gain

• Increased stamina – Athletes who exercise on an empty stomach have experienced more energy and stamina. It is believed that the combination of fasting and exercising triggers internal catalysts that force the breakdown of sugars and fat into energy, without sacrificing muscle mass.

• Helps with food cravings – As your Leptin and Ghrelin levels reset to your intermittent fasting schedule, old triggers to eat certain foods at certain times will be erased.

• Gene protection – Related to longevity and protection against diseases, including promising research on cancer

Chapter 4: Advantages of Intermittent Fasting

Intermittent fasting is becoming more and more popular as a weight-loss and health management tool. It has several important advantages over other approaches. Here are five of them.

1: Counting calories is unnecessary on intermittent fasting. Almost all dietary approaches involve counting calories. While this may be necessary following these short-term eating plans, it is almost impossible to do this long-term. This means that when the "diet" is over, the classical rebound fat gain is just around the corner after a period of rigidly controlling all food.

2: You don't have to go hungry on intermittent fasting. When you are eating all your daily calories in a window of several hours, it becomes much more difficult to overeat when compared to a traditional grazing approach. If you are fasting, you are not worrying about whether a snack is okay or not. Fasting is not eating, and when you break the fast, you eat if you are hungry. Simple!

3: Your body doesn't try to hang on to its fat stores when intermittent fasting. Most dietary approaches are necessarily restrictive. Your body is permanently deprived of enough food and reacts be going into starvation mode. It hangs on to all your fat stores and slows down your metabolism, exactly the opposite of what we want. However, when you can eat satisfaction as is the case on a fasting diet, your body responds by continuing to drop body fat.

4: An intermittent fasting diet is less restrictive than other diets. Let's be clear here if your idea of good food is a burger and fries; nothing is going to help you until you change your perception. However, it is perfectly possible and even helpful to have some leeway in what you eat. Sure, start with your protein and veggies, but some of what you like has some interesting and positive hormonal effects if you are trying to get lean or even build some muscle.

5: An intermittent fasting diet adapts to you. This is the real beauty of this approach. Instead of trying to find exactly the right number of grams of carbs or whatever at 10 am, you fit your daily fast to your life and goals. Some find a 16 hour fast from evening until the next day at lunch time works best. Others prefer a 24-hour cycle or even a 4-hour eating window. All of these are possible and have different advantages. It is a lifestyle rather than a diet.

Chapter 5: Intermittent Fasting Plan

The fact that many people have diverse demands makes it very challenging to give you an IF plan. Nonetheless, you can use the following guides to plan your program.

How Many Meals Will You Eat?

Whatever you like, factor it into your plan. Some would rather have one or two big meals during their eating window while some others may prefer to eat little meals all through the eating window. When Are You Working Out?

A regular exercise program is advised. However, you must factor this into your plan. Do you want to train on a full stomach or an empty one? It is usually better to have your meal after workouts because this way, the body can regain lost energy and the fuel needed for metabolism can be obtained from the meals.

Know Your Schedule.

Timing is the major focus of intermittent fasting and not particularly what you eat. For you to effectively do the IF plan, your eating period and cut-off time must be strictly adhered to. The eating and fasting windows usually control the lives of those involved in IF. They constantly have to check their time and plan accordingly.

Know Your Goals.

You should be aware of your calorie number, and how many calories you are to consume to maintain the caloric deficit of about 500 per day, that is if you want to adopt the IF plan. You are to keep a caloric surplus if you wish to build your body; however, all calories needed must be consumed during the eating window. It is harder to consume lots of calories because of the time frame by which you have to consume the food, but if you can consume a lot of calories, it is not likely that you will gain fat if you are in the intermittent fasting program.

You can continue eating what you are eating at the moment if you are okay with your weight level, just ensure your meals are consumed during the eating window. In other words, if you want to maintain your current weight but get healthier, keep the same calorie intake that you currently have but adopt the intermittent schedule.

Chapter 6: Getting Started with Intermittent Fasting

Instead of just jumping into fasting though I suggest you follow the information which will help you in forming a plan, sticking to the plan and finally getting the awesome results you want.

1. Decide a Starting Date.

I would highly suggest that you commence on a Monday. It just makes more sense. Pick a day and then follow the next few steps to be fully prepared for the starting time.

2. Choose a Fasting/Eating Split

Decide which eating and fasting window you want to adopt, again for beginners I always suggest the 16/8 as it is very easy to get used to and won't prove too difficult on your first attempt. Pick your window and then decide when you are going to stop eating the night before the fast – this will serve as your split, and for the first week, I suggest following it religiously. Once you've been practicing IF for a few weeks switching windows and times will become second nature to you, but for week 1 it's best to stick to the same times. So if you decide to stop eating at 9 pm on Sunday then you won't eat until 1 pm on Monday. After that 1-9pm will be your eating window.

3. Have a Cheat Day

The day before your first fast have a cheat day - eat a lot and eat whatever you want. This will serve two purposes for you. Firstly the more food you have in your system, the easier the first fast will be. Secondly, if you eat whatever you want the day before it means you won't crave these foods during the week.

4. Tell People

I highly suggest telling those who are closest to you to the new practice you are adopting. Explain why you are doing it and that you are committed – politely let them know you won't be eating at certain times and that you would love their support. By telling people in advance, you will offset the chances of them offering you foods when you fast.

5. Purchase Branch Chain Amino Acids

They are a pure form of protein and are unbelievably powerful if you are doing longer fasts. Consuming 10g of BCAAs will help curb hunger without breaking your fast. Do not take more than 10g per serving but feel free to have two servings during your fast. If you are going to be exercising, then I would highly suggest BCAAs.

6. Start

The most exciting part, you get to start, take action and see results. No matter how much you read or research the most important thing is taking action, nothing else will get you in shape.

Chapter 7: Tips to Manage Hunger

Some of the ways to keep the hunger under control are:

Meditation

Meditation helps you to relax, sit still and control how you think- this can help control anxiety and stress. Although this is not the easiest way to control hunger, meditation works miracles over time. As you get better at it, you will learn to control hunger and even perhaps embrace it.

Meditating will help you avoid the temptations of breaking a fast as you get to think clearly of what you want and the benefits you will get after sticking to the fast.

Have a cup of coffee or organic tea

Other than water, other fluids can help keep the hunger as far from you as possible. Caffeine and other stimulants of the nervous system work as appetite suppressants; consumption of coffee has been proven to stimulate the release of the hormone cholecystokinin (CCK) which is one of the hormones released after eating that gives us a calm feeling. This hormone makes us full and takes away the feelings of eating.

Also, a simple cup of tea or coffee can hydrate your system and boost your energy levels with a bonus of delivering a wave of antioxidants. Start your day with a cup of either (tea or coffee) or have a cup whenever you feel hunger kicking in.

Drinking lots of water

Aside from being the healthiest and easiest method of fighting hunger, staying well hydrated can make fasting much easier to get through. Most of the time, thirst is confused for hunger so anytime you feel hungry, just gobble down a glass of water. Keep this in mind as it will be your number 1 way to stave off hunger.

Play some sports or engage in a hobby

Any physical activity that you engage in is going to have a positive impact on your fast- just as long as you keep it moderate. If you have favorite sport such as basketball or tennis or any other type of physical hobby such as boxing, then engage in it during the fasting period.

Engage in some short and intense exercise

Engaging in intervals of short and intense exercise during the fasting period is a sure way to keep your mind from focusing on hunger. Intense exercise such as sprinting or lifting weights also blasts fats and boosts muscles and more importantly, directly suppresses appetite.

Different types of exercises can lead to production or reduction of different kinds of appetite suppressing hormones.

If you are not at work, then go crazy on household chores

If your fast day falls on a day when you are not at work, then household chores will do the trick when it comes to fighting off hunger.

Do any pending work-related tasks

Do you know that report or project that you have been putting off or all those unread emails that are packed in your inbox? This is the great opportunity to work on them. Ensure that your fast is productive and that you don't spend the whole day obsessing over your next meal.

When you are not eating, base your focus on something else productive- it could be school work, job-related tasks or related social activities. The busier you are, the more successful you're fast will be.

Munch on some live foods

This should be the last option for controlling hunger. If you find out that you simply cant 100% control your hunger and you need to eat then the best option is to enter into a 'controlled fast'- this is similar to the undereating phase of the warrior diet.

Here, you will have to eat very lightly during the fast- foods that have the lowest glycemic index. The foods should only be live veggies and fruits- they should not be cooked at all. Also, make sure to keep the servings small.

Take a walk

Taking brisk walks increases fat burning effects of a fast. A brisk walk also nourishes a healthy heart and promotes general health. Combining a fast and a brisk walk could be the best thing you could do for your body.

Like other kinds of exercise, a brisk walk can keep your hunger in control. It can do this by first of all providing a fun distraction and motivating the body to start burning stored fat for energy.

Chapter 8: Common Mistakes associated with Intermittent Fasting

Your Reasons Aren't Strong Enough

As stated earlier, you need to come up with several compelling reasons to implement Intermittent Fasting into your life. If you don't have enough reasons that emotionally compel you at all times, you will be more likely to fail. Also, there is a chance that people will question your decision and if you aren't able to fully explain to yourself exactly why you need to implement Intermittent Fasting, at some point you will think: "Why bother? Screw this."

Going Too Hard

Fasting diet. Why? Because you are trying to implement all the habits at once. While I understand that you want to implement Intermittent Fasting into your life quickly, it isn't the smartest way to go about it. We as human beings have a limited amount of willpower, and every time you try to implement a new habit, you use up a bit.

So, you can understand that if you try to implement them all at once, you will deplete all of your willpower very quickly. When this happens, you have reached your breaking point. When you have reached your breaking point, you will most likely give up on Intermittent Fasting and go back to doing things the old way. Or worse, you there will be a chance that you will develop bad habits.

Too Many Distractions from people

The first thing you need to realize is that it isn't their fault that you aren't succeeding with Intermittent Fasting. It is just that your and their goals conflict. A way to get around this is by asking them if they want to help you with the issue. Explain to them why Intermittent Fasting is so important to you and show them what results it brings you. Ask them if they can respect your decision and whether they can eat at different moments if you are around.

Eliminate all distractions. As stated earlier, you need to come up with several compelling reasons to implement Intermittent Fasting into your life. If you don't have enough reasons that emotionally compel you at all times, you will be more likely to fail.

Chapter 9: Intermittent Fasting for Consistent Weight Loss

Intermittent fasting involves alternating your eating pattern between periods of fasting (consuming only water) and non-fasting (eating). The eating times can be highly variable and extend over several days. Some of the longer non-eating periods include a 36-hour fast followed by 12 hours of eating (usually broken into 3 meals about 3-4 hours apart) Most intermittent fasting diets extend over a 24-hour period, allowing the person to stay consistent from day to day. The more aggressive of these day-long fasts limit a person to 4 hours of eating (usually at night). The most widely accepted fasting regimen involves an 8-hour window for eating.

Intermittent fasting has been studied extensively on both animals and humans. Unless the fast was extended beyond 36 hours, no negative effects were observed in the test subjects (other than mild to moderate hunger pains). Intermittent fasting has been shown to decrease body fat, stabilize blood sugars, and increase muscle response.

How does it work? It all revolves around the hormone insulin. Your body releases insulin whenever you consume food (more so for foods high in carbohydrates). The insulin stimulates the absorption of nutrients (mostly glucose) into your fat and muscle tissue. Since most of the time, the muscle cells are not energy deprived, excess nutrients after meals are stored in your fat tissue (glucose is also stored as glycogen in your liver). It takes about 3 hours after meal times before your body's insulin level drops to pre-meal levels. At the lower insulin concentrations, your liver and fat tissue release the stored glucose and fatty acids into your bloodstream for energy. By extending the time between meals, you increase the length of this catabolic state when your body burns off fat.

Were you told to eat 5-6 small meals each day? Frequent meal consumption hinders the body's fat-burning process. Under a similar diet, a person using an intermittent fasting approach will attain a lower body fat percentage than the frequent eater. Keep in mind, however, that the quality of your diet is more important than the timing. Intermittent fasting is not an excuse for binging on junk food later at night. You still need to eat clean. Furthermore, you will want to increase your protein consumption when on a fasting diet. Protein is the best macronutrient regarding satiety, meaning that calorie-for-calorie, protein will subdue the feeling of hunger for longer than will carbohydrates or fats. Eating a high-protein/low-carb diet is a must, especially on non-workout days.

Chapter 10: Intermittent Fasting on Heart Disease and Diabetes

Intermittent fasting with water might just bring down your heart disease risks and chances of developing diabetes. The research was conducted in an area where up to 65% of the population are Mormons who, in observance of their faith, fast one day every month.

Interesting that heart disease rates are consistently lowest in this area. Until recently, many experts attributed this to the fact the Mormon Church discourages smoking by members. However, even though the number of smokers has decreased across the U.S., Utah continues to have a heart disease rate that is lower than the rest.

In earlier work, the same research team found that subjects who answered "yes" when asked whether they fasted had less heart disease. The latest study sought to reproduce and take these earlier results further, to see if this might be the reason for the lower heart disease risk.

In an accompanying study, the researchers examined blood markers for heart risks in those who hadn't fasted over the last 12 hours. The markers were reviewed when the subjects fasted and also monitored during a normal day of eating. The fasts were water only, though participants were allowed to take medication.

During the fast, the levels of good cholesterol (HDL) rose, as did LDL (bad) cholesterol and total cholesterol numbers - not favorable to be sure, but the researchers believe the rise may be temporary. But, those fasting also had reductions in dangerous blood fats known as triglycerides, as well as blood sugar levels. When you fast, the body tries to preserve its cells and tissue, using fats instead of sugars for fuel.

There are lots of questions to answer before anyone will suggest fasting as a treatment for heart disease. Researchers do know that those who fast have a lower incidence of diabetes and heart disease, but just how this works will need more study before we can say for certain.

You've probably heard about fasts... juice fasts are popular on the internet. But comparing water only fast to juice fast is not a fair comparison. While they might provide a benefit to your heart, as shown in animal studies, the benefit is not as great as the water only fasting.

You should also know that fasting isn't for everyone. Young children, pregnant or nursing mothers and those with certain health conditions should not do this. One of the other dangers is that a fast might prompt binge eating that destroys any health benefits you might have gotten.

Some researchers would like to point out that while not eating will decrease certain numbers, doing something to the extreme is not always the best choice.

What you eat, has far more impact on your heart disease risks than a single day event. Another thing, intermittent fasting isn't a magic potion or silver bullet... it's a lifestyle choice that becomes a part of your life. Not just for a while, but over the long term.

Chapter 11: Who is supposed to Fast and who is not

People who currently eat an unhealthy diet:

People who eat a good deal of fast food, processed foods, and sugar can benefit from the Intermittent Fast Diet's nutritionally balanced approach. The focus of both fasting and non- fasting days is on whole foods: primarily lean meats, fresh fruits and vegetables, low-fat dairy, and whole grains. Many people find that after eating this type of diet for a few weeks, they are better able to appreciate healthier whole foods and have a better understanding of what makes a well-rounded diet.

People Who Are Well-Suited for the Intermittent Fast Diet

The Intermittent Fast Diet can be a great plan for anyone who is otherwise healthy but would like to lose weight and shed body fat. However, the format of the diet can make it especially beneficial to some specific groups of people.

People who are addicted to sugary foods or empty calories:

Many people become addicted to sugary foods, high-carbohydrate processed snacks, and empty calorie beverages such as sodas and blended coffee drinks, which have lots of calories and little to no nutrition. For some of these people, the Intermittent Fast Diet can have the added benefit of helping them break those addictions. This is not only because of the focus on whole foods but also because of the calorie restrictions on fasting days. When you only have 500 to 600 calories to use in a day, it's hard to justify spending half of it on one cola. After a week or two of living without those foods, many people report that the cravings and withdrawal symptoms subside.

People Who Are Not Good Candidates for the Intermittent Fast Diet

People with type 2 diabetes should not undertake this diet. Although some evidence shows that it may correct imbalances of or insensitivity to insulin, once type 2 diabetes has been diagnosed, fasting is not advised.

In particular, women who are pregnant or nursing should not attempt intermittent fasting. The calorie guidelines for the fasting days are simply too low. However, once you have had your baby and have finished nursing, intermittent fasting can help you get your pre-pregnancy body back.

People who need an especially simple plan:

Some people just naturally do better when steps and choices are very limited. A diet with too many variations and choices or that requires too much planning and decision- making are often hard for such people to maintain. The Intermittent Fast Diet is simple, straightforward, and mapped out step by step. Because of calorie limitations, the fasting day meal plans are extremely simple, and recipes often have just a few ingredients.

Children and adolescents should not go on the Intermittent Fast Diet. Please consult a pediatrician or nutritionist if you are seeking a weight-loss plan for anyone under eighteen years of age.

Chapter 12: Questions About Intermittent Fasting

Is an Intermittent Fasting Diet the Right Choice For Me?

It is important to realize that the key is nutrition and finding an approach that works for you long-term. This is where an intermittent fasting diet is a particularly interesting option when compared to other dietary approaches.

So does an intermittent fasting diet work when compared to other diets? The answer here is a resounding yes. For example, using a 16 hour fast will keep your body burning fat for most of every day! And getting all of your calories during a relatively small eating window stops your body from going into starvation mode and desperately hanging onto body-fat. Compared to a normal reduced calorie diet, this is a huge difference. While any reduced calorie approach will initially lead to fat-loss, your body is an efficient machine and will compensate by slowing down your metabolism (the exact opposite of what you want) and holding onto body fat.

Is an intermittent fasting diet restrictive? Any diet, by its very nature, involves making better food choices. If someone tries to sell you on the pancake diet, run a mile! Eating rubbish can never be a good choice. However, most diets will have you try to eat clean all the time. This is very hard to do and is directly linked to finding yourself eating 12 doughnuts in one sitting after a couple of weeks of deprivation! Intermittent fasting also involves healthy food choices, but it does give you more wiggle room. It is difficult to eat to much junk in a small eating window after you have already had your healthy food. It does let you eat enough to stop you falling off the wagon, however.

Perhaps the real advantage of intermittent fasting is that it can be a lifestyle rather than a short-term approach. With most diets, even if you do manage to follow it long enough to get results tend to be followed by a rebound-that is a return to poor eating and fat gain. By viewing fasting as a long-term solution, this problem effectively disappears.

Should I take vitamins when I intermittently fast?

It is more important than ever to take vitamins and supplements when fasting, as you are skipping meals that were helping to supply you with these vital nutrients and it's important that you replace them. The biggest problem with vitamins and fasting is that taking a vitamin pill in a fasted state may result in stomach pain, nausea, and diarrhea. To avoid these unpleasant, unsettling effects, try and get your vitamins down while in the fed state. If this is impossible, try taking your vitamins at night so you can sleep through the discomfort.

Alternatively, you might choose vitamins in liquid form, as they are easier to digest while fasting. If you don't normally take vitamins, a basic multivitamin that provides 100% of your daily intake is a great start to ensure you aren't missing out on anything while intermittently fasting.

Why would anyone fast who doesn't want to lose weight?

It may seem odd to someone who is considering intermittently fasting to lose weight, for anyone who has their weight under control to change their eating habits or patterns. After all, aren't they already living the dream? Let's not forget about all the other benefits of intermittent fasting:

- Fasting for health benefits: Some people swear by fasting because they feel it improves their sleep, mental clarity, and helps them control and maintain chronic diseases such as diabetes, cardiovascular disease, multiple sclerosis, fibromyalgia, chronic fatigue syndrome, cancer and the side effects from chemotherapy.

- Fasting for athletes: Fasting offers a consistent method of fueling and resting the body that works under many of the same principles as training and rest days. It offers them a much more convenient way to ensure that they consume the food they need to train than the other option of eating small meals every 2 or 3 hours, and it allows them to maintain a nutrition routine that provides a lengthier feeding time which can be enjoyed with friends and family.

- Fasting for busy people with poor eating habits: People who travel a lot for business often end up feeling less than well most of the time, due to poor eating habits developed as a result of airport restaurants and late-night vending machines.

- Make sure you are well-hydrated and avoid salty or sugary foods before you fast.

- Don't stuff yourself the night before you fast. This "last supper" mentality is a rookie mistake that will give you indigestion, a poor night's sleep, and an even ruder awakening to your stomach and brain when you follow up the preceding evening's bacchanalia with a fasting period.

Why do I get headaches when I fast and how can I stop them?

Complaints of headaches especially when beginning an intermittent fasting program are quite common. If you are waking with a headache, you may not have hydrated yourself enough the night before. Not drinking enough water is one of the biggest culprits of headaches during fasting and water should be imbibed throughout the fasting/feeding process. Headaches can also be a side effect of the detoxing process that occurs in intermittent fasting and will be especially prevalent in the beginning stages of incorporating the program into your health regime.

Isn't intermittent fasting just a fancy way of saying I'm starving myself?

• Fatty acids are used by the body as an energy source for muscles but lower the amount of glucose that travels to the brain. Fatty acids also include a chemical called glycerol that can be used, like glucose as an energy source, but it too will eventually run out.

• Fat stores are depleted, and the body turns to stored protein for energy, breaking down muscle tissue. The muscle tissue breaks down very quickly. When all sources of protein are gone, cells can no longer function.

• The body does not have the energy to fight off bacteria and viruses. It takes 8 to 12 weeks to starve to death, although there have been cases of people surviving 25 weeks or more.

Is intermittent fasting safe for women?

Women are more hormonally sensitive than men. Because of this, they may respond more intensely to the challenges of intermittent fasting and need to consult with a medical professional before starting an intermittent fasting program, especially if they have menstrual and fertility issues. Once intermittent fasting has been undertaken, women should also pay special attention to their menstrual cycle, and seek medical guidance if they begin missing periods.

There is a modified technique of intermittent fasting that will help women who experience hormonal sensitivity. This is a more progressive approach that will help the female body adapt to fasting.

• Fast for 12-16 hours

• On fasting days, stick to light workouts such as yoga or light cardio

• Fast on 2-3 nonconsecutive days per week

• After a few weeks, add another day of fasting and monitor how it goes.

• Drink loads of water

• Save strength training for feeding periods or feeding days

Why can't I have a protein shake when I'm fasting?

You can't eat food when you are intermittently fasting – hence you can't drink a protein shake. People get confused about protein shakes – check out diet, fitness, and nutrition and health websites if you don't believe me. I used to shake my head in wonder when I first saw this question asked.

If you are on a 5:2 type of intermittent fasting program and you are consuming 500 to 600 calories on your "low" days, feel free to indulge in one or 2 of these shakes if they don't bring you over your total calorie count. If you are on Whole Day Fasting or in the fasting portion of your Time Restricted intermittent fasting cycle, don't even think about it!

How can I fast when I'm on vacation?

I indirectly referred to the answer to this question when I was explaining some of the advantages of Whole Day Fasting and 5:2 Intermittent Fasting. Because you are confining your fasting to 2 non-consecutive days of the week, you can automatically end up with a 4-day feeding unit of time. This will help the eating challenges of holidays and vacations in a big way.

Conclusion

Thank you again for downloading this book!

I hope this book was able to help you to know more about intermittent fasting.

When engaged in intermittent fasting, your body flourishes when you follow the cyclical approach to ingestion and digestion. As beneficial as skipping occasional meals can be, especially in the morning, fasting which occurs early in the morning till late in the afternoon and feasting which occurs from late in the afternoon till night may help with body detoxification, improve your immune functions, and also encourage the burning of body fat. You need to know everything to do with intermittent fasting, as individuals with a shallow knowledge of IF can be confused.

History shows that intermittent fasting is a popular act amongst religious individuals, such as Christians and Muslims. Lent, during which Christians practice fasting, is a bit different from intermittent fasting, although they do abstain from food, abstain from leisurely acts or anything that gives them pleasure, and consecrate themselves for a common cause to purify themselves as a worthy living sacrifice. For forty days, Christians abstain from anything that is termed as corrupt, according to their religious beliefs.

For Muslims, a specific period is dedicated to fasting, which is referred to as the month of Ramadan. During this time, Muslims engage in the practice of total abstinence during the day from food, drinks, and sexual activity. Muslims consecrate themselves from sunrise to sunset all throughout the month of Ramadan.

Remember, I told you that intermittent fasting could be extreme and tough if you do not understand all that needs to be understood about it.

The next step is to evaluate if you able to do intermittent fasting.

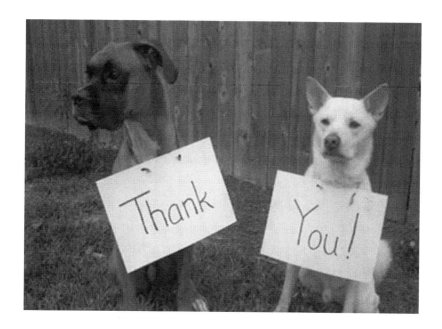

Finally, if you enjoyed this book, then I'd like to ask you for a favor, would you be kind enough to leave a review for this book on Amazon? It'd be greatly appreciated!

Thank you and good luck!

Made in the USA
Lexington, KY
11 May 2018